THE INTERMITTENT FASTING 16/8 LIFESTYLE

How I Lost 10 Lbs. In A Month While
Still Eating All My Favorite Foods

By

Jasmine Carter

Table of Contents

Introduction

Most people would agree that dieting is stressful, there are too many diet options, and most diets are not sustainable, leaving them to believe losing or maintaining weight is impossible. What if I told you I knew a way for you to successfully eat the meals that you desire and eat your absolute favorite foods, when you wanted too, in the easiest and fastest way, and still lose weight and/or maintain weight depending on your meal choices? Would you be interested? Ok, great. In this book, you will learn how to change your eating habits to accommodate a new lifestyle to allow you to lose weight and/or maintain weight loss. This new habit and lifestyle change is called Intermittent Fasting.

Some advantages of this lifestyle are as follows: there is no food group that must be excluded, you can select your meals and when to eat, there are no types of purchases that must be made, you will see a spike in your energy level, and more.

It was only 483 days ago that I and my wife was considered obese and were unable to conceive. Together and individually, we had tried many of the available options to include: Adkins Diet, Keto Diet, Low Carb Diet, No Sugar Diet, No Meat Diet, Vegan Diet, Weight Watchers, Raw Food Diet, and more. Because of this new lifestyle change, together we successfully lost over 160 lbs. and have maintained the weight loss for over a year and are now proud parents of a baby boy. This lifestyle change made it easy for us to adapt, and as a bonus of losing and maintaining this weight loss, we were able to naturally conceive.

By continuing to read this book, you will have all the tools to lose weight and maintain that weight loss in one place. This book explains the lifestyle change, how it works, and the science behind how it works. It also documents details on how to set up your new lifestyle, key information to know before starting, best tips for beginners, an actual daily protocol, how to monitor your progress, how to deal with setbacks, and much more! These and more details have proven a success; this book will ensure a lifestyle change and give you complete weight management. Start today, you can lose 10 pounds in the first week and keep it off forever!

The Power of Intermittent Fasting

What is Fasting? Intermittently?

Fasting is a choice to abstain from eating and/or drinking for a period. Intermittent Fasting is an eating lifestyle, in which you only eat during a specific feeding window, and not consume calories during your fasting window. A feeding window is a time in which you have decided to intake calories. A fasting window is a time in which you have decided NOT to consume calories.

Intermittent Fasting, or "IF", is the process of choosing a feeding window and a fasting window that equals 24 hours in your day. This is a lifestyle choice that does not rely on food restrictions like other types of diet tactics. Intermittent Fasting is popular today because it is now associated with weight management and weight loss and offers many benefits without much effort besides deciding and committing to the feeding and fasting windows that you have chosen. [1] There are multiple methods in which people choose to fast, sometimes by hours, sometimes by days, sometimes by meals. The emphasis here will be on the basic feeding/fasting windows in a daily hourly method.

Intermittent Fasting 16:8 Method

The Intermittent Fasting 16:8 Method is when you fast 16 hours out of the day, and only eat during a total of 8 hours a day. The fasting window is a total of 16 hours a day; Your fasting window will mostly be during the time you are sleeping. During your fasting window, you will NOT consume ANY calories at all. Not eating when your mind and body are accustomed to eating will be difficult, but the challenge is mind over matter, and you matter, so you will succeed. Choose a time to start and stop your feeding window, when the feeding window stops, the fasting window starts, and when the fasting window stops, the feeding window starts, and so on.

The Benefits & Why the 16:8 Method

Intermittent Fasting is not complicated, and it does not have to affect the way you live your daily life. This lifestyle will compliment your current life and not work against it. You will still be able to enjoy dinner with your family, happy hour with your friends, and a drink after dinner if you want. Living this lifestyle, there is no predetermined time that must be used as the feeding and/or fasting window, this is your choice; the fasting and feeding times can be set according to your current personal schedule.

With the other diets, you must exclude carbs, sugars, meats, alcohol, social outings, your wants, flavors, fats, and/or more, but with IF you DO NOT have to exclude a food group if you do not choose to. Other diet tactics, take too much mental space to keep up; there are way too many food restrictions and rules. With the 16:8 method, some people even consume fewer calories, and sometimes fewer meals, than they plan to because you are only eating during your 8-hour feeding window and you are accustomed to eating more or longer hours in a day.

With this method, you do not have to eat breakfast, but you can eat breakfast if you want at whatever time you choose. Breakfast is considered the first meal of the day and has always been recognized as the most important meal of the day, you can still have this meal, it may just be at a different time than the average person considers breakfast time. Your breakfast, lunch, and dinner times may be at average times if you want or they can be non-traditional times, this is again your choice when living an IF lifestyle. You do not have to stop eating by 6pm, 7pm, or 8pm; You stop eating when your feeding window is over, based on the time you have chosen.

There are no supplements or disgusting shakes or drinks that you are required to ingest at certain times a day every day. There are no books or journals or apps you must purchase or carry around with you to have to keep track of your meals, or the calories, or macros, or carbs, etc. You are not required to increase your spending in any way to start or maintain an IF lifestyle, which is the ultimate advantage of living this lifestyle. Any person with any income with any type of career and schedule can use the 16:8 method of intermittent fasting.

Some people struggle with food cravings, emotional eating habits, food addictions and triggers, binge eating, food obsessiveness, and more. These habits could be physiological or psychological, depends on the individual. Physiological eating habits are healthier and the end goal. Psychological eating habits are displayed in a person when they have eaten and are physically full, there is no actual physical hunger pains or needs at that time, but they still eat more for innumerable reasons in their head.

The first week or so of this lifestyle change to Intermittent Fasting could help people recognize the differences between physical hunger and psychological hunger.

Leangains Method

The 16:8 Method is also known as the Leangains Method, coined by Martin Berkhan. This is a high protein eating lifestyle, which is focused on carb, fat, and protein ratio, these are called your macronutrients. The Leangains Method or protocol also promotes exercise heavily.

On workout days, the largest meal of the day should be the post-workout meal. It consists of high carbs, moderate proteins, and low fat. On non-work out days, the largest meal should be the first meal of the day, and because there is no workout that day the calorie intake should be less, the fat intake should be higher, along with fibrous veggies, meat, and fruit as the components of this meal, there should be little to no carb intake. Dinner, the last meal of each day, should consist of slow digesting protein options like eggs, fish, nut butter, dairy, and more. These types of food before bed keeps the body nourished during sleep and the fasted state. [10]

How does IF Work?

This type of fasting is NOT all hype with no context; there is science behind the efficacy of intermittent fasting on human health. There are many health benefits, in addition to weight loss and/or weight management, as discussed previously. Blood pressure, triglycerides, fat mass, blood glucose, LDL cholesterol, and blood sugars all improve, as intermittent fasting becomes more and more familiar within your body system. [2]

Intermittent fasting has been associated with diabetes prevention and has resulted in the reprieve of pre-diabetic symptoms. Sugar is what our cells use for energy. If our cells don't use it for energy, the sugar is stored as fat within our fat cells. Sugar can only enter our cells with insulin. Insulin is what brings sugar into our fat cells and keeps it there. Intermittent Fasting lowers insulin levels, which prevents our fat cells from holding on to stored sugar in our bodies, which inevitably, if not released, causes a decrease in energy. The longer a person fasts, the more fat cells your body will burn for fuel instead of storing as body fat, which will result in increased energy. [12]

Intermittent fasting also significantly improves insulin sensitivity. Insulin sensitivity describes how sensitive the body is to the effects of insulin; having a good sensitivity to insulin is a sign of good health. Intermittent Fasting drops your insulin levels, which alters your body's demand for insulin in a good way, it also resets your insulin sensitivity.[3] Of lately, intermittent fasting has been associated with preserving memory and learning functionality; once your body starts using its fat stores for energy, ketones are then used, which is what protects the neurons for memory and learning functions.[4,15]

Like with exercise, Intermittent fasting puts your bodies cells under mild stress. A physiological benefit of intermittent fasting is that your body learns to cope with this stress and fight back, hence resist disease more and more as your body learns to cope. This fasting is associated with making your bodies overall health stronger. Intermittent Fasting is reportedly been associated with an influence on metabolic regulations, this includes circadian rhythm, gut microbes, and modifiable lifestyle behaviors.

Humans have evolved to perform most physiological processes at optimal times; certain activities are optimally done during the day hours and others, like sleep, are done at night, this is what most people call natural. A circadian rhythm is the regular recurrence of life activities in a 24-hour cycle. Consuming food outside of the normal feed phase, which is during the night hours when people should be sleep, resets some circadian rhythms and disrupts energy balance; hence a major effect on a persons metabolism. Any fasting that encourages NOT eating during the night hours allowing the body to burn fatter, synchronizes food intake with the optimal times to eat. [2, 16]

Having an intermittent fasting lifestyle seems to have a positive impact on gut microbiota. Gut microbiota is a complex community of microorganisms that live in your digestive tract. This positivity also goes along with the circadian rhythms. Gastric emptying and blood flow function optimally during the daytime rather than at night, so disturbing circadian may negatively affect gastrointestinal functions and ultimately impair metabolism and health.[3]

Intermittent fasting has improved self-reported sleep satisfaction. Night time eating has been associated with sleep deprivation and insomnia, which can have negative effects on insulin resistance. Insulin resistance increases the risk of Diabetes and other cardiovascular diseases. The increased effects of prolonged nightly fasting can prevent Diabetes, other cardiovascular diseases, negative insulin resistance, insomnia, and/or sleep deprivation. [1]

The Protocol

Preparing for a Lifestyle Change

How to Start (Setting up Fasting and Feeding Times)

To get started all you need is a good idea of your daily routine schedule, on average, as each day is not created equal for sure. Think back and jot down the time frame in which you think you do most of your eating on an average day. Next, jot down the time in which you think you get the most sleep. Lastly, jot down other important time frames that are important to your average daily routine. Some important time frames I jotted down and considered initially were happy hours with my spouse and friends, and family dinner time, in which we eat dinner together each day.

I considered that on average, my eating times ranged from 10:00 AM to about 8:00 PM on weekdays and from 12:00 PM to midnight on the weekends, as I have a great social life. With terrible sleeping habits, I was sleeping around midnight, waking up at 8:00 AM at the latest on weekdays and from 2:00 AM to 12:00 PM on weekends.

Review your notes and decide on the best 8 hours out of your day to be considered your feeding window. With this schedule, I would say a good starting feeding window would be 12:00 PM to 8:00 PM daily. With this feeding window, the fasting window would automatically be daily starting at 8:00 PM and fast until 12:00 PM. Some people consume 3 meals during this 8-hour window, but I found that to be impossible for me, so I consume 2 moderate portioned sized meals and eat snacks at other times during the feeding window. You can decide to eat how many meals and snacks you want while intermittent fasting, but decide and be consistent.

Meal Planning

Meal planning, also known as meal prep, is NOT required to be successful with intermittent fasting, however, it does a good job of preparing you for even more success with your feeding window. Meal prep is preparing some or all meals/snacks in advance to have on hand when needed. Meal prep saves you time, so you aren't preparing meals/snacks each day and it takes away the thought process of what you will eat during your feeding windows daily. By meal prepping, there is less room for failure, especially for beginners. With meal planning comes the bonus of preparing healthier options to eat during your feeding window, instead of choosing quickly processed and prepacked options because it's convenient.

For me there are many steps to Meal Planning. Meal Planning consists of creating full meals (this includes recipes), creating all-inclusive grocery lists, reviewing your own kitchen to see what you already have and what you need, then altering your grocery list, and finally going grocery shopping.

Creating meals takes creativity. With the world wide web, there are plenty of recipes and meals ideas for available options. Being creative means not always eating the same thing day in and day out. Change up your breakfast options, lunch options, dinner options, and snacks. Season the food differently. Cook a different cut of the beef. Garnish it differently. Make it a soup or salad instead of a casserole. Make vegetables a snack in some way. Find ways to increase your protein intake. Add more green leaves to your protein shakes and/or more vegetables or fruits. Decide on 2-3 lunch and dinner options, and 2-3 snack options.

Once you have decided on what meals you have created and the recipes, you will need to search through your kitchen cabinets, freezer, pantry, and refrigerator to see what you have already have and don't need to purchase when you go food shopping. This includes everything, meats, sides, fresh vegetables, fresh fruit, drinks, snack options, spices, herbs, oils, breads, wraps, and more. Revise your grocery shopping list to include what you need.

Proceed to go to the grocery stores and pick up the items on your list. In preparation for meal prep. Meal prep is taking all of your groceries and cutting up everything that needs to be cut up, washing everything that needs to be washed, marinating everything that needs to be marinated, seasoning everything that needs to be seasoned, baking everything that needs to be backed, cooking everything that needs to be cooked, measure everything that needs to be measured to the appropriate portion, and packing it all in individual meal Tupperware containers to easily grab and go when needed. Although highly recommended, meal planning and prep, is NOT required for intermittent fasting.

Portion Control, Food Labels, & Measurements

Portion control is NOT necessarily required when intermittent fasting, however, because you are not restricting any food groups and you can technically eat what you want during your feeding window, portion control becomes even more important than meal prep, but could also work in speeding up the weight loss when treated equally. Portion control does not mean you have to eat tiny portions of everything. Portion control is the serving size on the label or the amount that is generally served. To best practice portion control when your meal prep, measure your foods and package them into the containers before storing them away for later meals. Another tip to use, to ensure you are eating proportionately, is to drink a glass of water to ensure you are hungry and not just thirsty and to ensure you do not overeat.

Food Labels displays the nutrient content/nutritional facts, calories, and serving sizes for packaged foods. Reading food labels will ensure you are not eating too much at one time, this is fundamentally portion control at its best. The first things to review is the serving size. Serving size is the portion size that is generally served at once. The calorie count displays how many calories are in one serving. Food labels also include the total fats, cholesterol, sodium, and total carbohydrates per serving size. Additionally, the % daily value displays how much this serving will count towards your daily intake, try not to go over 100% in any category. Reading and understanding food labels are NOT required to be successful while intermittent fasting, but this could enhance results.

Counting net carbs is another big topic of discussion that people tend to gravitate too. To count net carbs, subtract the dietary fiber from the total carbohydrates count, this equals net carbs. Counting net carbs only is an acceptable way to eat and meal plan, BUT counting net carbs is not required to intermittent fast. Counting net carbs and calories are NOT required for intermittent fasting. [17]

Measuring foods is NOT necessarily required when intermittent fasting, but it ensures you are not eating too much of whatever you choose to eat. Use smaller containers to ensure you are eating a good amount of food to be full, but not stuffed. Never eat from the package that the snack came in, and limit distractions while you eat, as people usually overeat while doing activities, such as watching television. Measuring food is important for portion control, but not required for intermittent fasting.

Choose Food Options Wisely/Balanced Options

When following an intermittent fasting lifestyle, you are not restricted from any food group and you can choose your own meal options, BUT food choices are still (as always) important. It is important to have good nutrition that emphasizes a diet that provides a complete source of minerals, vitamins, and nutrients for the healthiest functioning body.

A diet is considered the sum of all foods eaten, but it refers to the use of specific intake of nutrition. Any healthy diet should include whole and unprocessed foods over processed and/or liquid foods to include plenty of fruits and vegetables, lean proteins, some fats and oils, and grains; this would be considered a balanced meal, these are also called energy-dense foods. Energy-dense foods are high in fiber and helps to retain natural water. [14]

When fasting, try to eat more non-starchy vegetables and lean proteins. Choose foods that are whole grain and stay away from refined grains and flours. Fruit is going to be the best option to try to curb the still existing sweet tooth, especially for beginners. Choose a non-dairy over dairy and eat fats and oils in moderation and choose the healthiest forms of fats and oils.

Fresh fruits and vegetables are favored over frozen and canned, but any vegetable is better than no vegetables at all. Choose lean cuts of protein and to increase your protein intake add vegetarian sources, like beans and soy products. Try almond, soy, or cashew non-dairy options to limit your dairy intake, as dairy is one of the world's leading allergens. Other leading allergens include eggs, peanuts, and shellfish. [1] Make carbs toppers instead of the base of your meals. When buying pasta, bread, crackers, and more always look for whole grain listed as the first ingredient on the nutrition label. Eat half of an avocado at least once a day to increase your healthy fat intake.

According to the USDA, there are 5 principle guidelines to follow to satisfy your dietary needs. Follow a healthy eating pattern across your entire lifespan, a lot of people are not following this first guideline. An eating pattern is your liquids and foods intake and your routine way of eating. Following this first guideline ensures nutrient adequacy, healthy body systems, and lower risks to chronic disease invasions of your body. The second and fourth guideline is to focus on the amount of food and liquids you consume and to be focused on eating nutrient-dense foods from all the major food groups and how to shift from bad choices to good choices. The decisions you make are most important. You are the important link that makes the difference, you are in control of ensuring you are meeting these guidelines. Meeting these guidelines is the responsibility of all people.

The third guideline is to limit the number of calories that do not come from nutrient-dense foods, such as added sugars, high sodium, and trans and saturated fats. According to the USDA, healthy eating meals consist of a whole fruit, fresh vegetables, dairy, protein, whole grains, and oils. The fifth guideline is teaching you how to share your knowledge with others; it states that support is necessary for change for everyone and that it is all our jobs to support healthy eating habits. [1]

Physical Activity

Like meal planning, measuring foods, reading food labels, and portion control, exercise is NOT required, but beneficial to your overall results while intermittent fasting. The American Heart Association recommends some form of physical activity for at least 30 minutes daily. [13]

Create a workout schedule. Make a leg day, an arms day, cardio day, total body weight day, and more. A schedule starts to make you more consistent and accountable. On days when you feel unmotivated to do one you have the other. If you are already exercise, intermittent fasting can only improve your results. The combination of intermittent fasting and exercise maximizes weight loss and/or weight maintenance.

Mindset

The biggest barrier, if any, will be your mindset. The barrier will be the already set attitudes and assumptions you have in your head specifically as it relates to the relationship you have with food and eating food. Think mind over matter, and you matter the most to yourself, so take better care of yourself. To sustain following an intermittent lifestyle, you will need to erase or ignore all prior assumptions or attitudes related to diets/lifestyle changes, losing weight, current food habits, current eating schedules, change in general, and more. Once started, try to make optimal choices for you and be disciplined in being consistent in carrying plans throughout. To be successful you will need to think and act differently for optimal results.

Surviving Longer While Hungry

Hunger is feeling uncomfortable and/or being weak due to a lack of food. Hunger can be physical, but it can also just be a desire or want rather than a need right at that moment. The body sometimes responds as if its hunger, but sometimes we are thirsty and are yearning for liquids and not food, therefore your water intake is imperative to your success in extending to longer fasting windows.

To habituate longer fasting windows and/or to resist food during your fasting window to make it to the feeding window, staying productive is vital. Stay busy by any means necessary. It is a great idea to exercise during this time or stay busy with your professional or personal work. Being lazy and feeling bored are false indicators to your body that you may be hungry when really you are just in a slump or bored. The more you think about food the weaker your body thinks your mind is and eventually this will be your takedown.

Frequently Asked Questions for Beginners

Most types of changes come with a lot of questions, intermittent fasting is no different. Here are some frequently asked questions from beginners: How should I schedule my feeding and fasting times if I work overnight or long shifts? Schedule your feeding and fasting window according to your own time, which means your feeding window would be more so evenings and overnight and the fasting more of the daytime when you are sleeping.

Can I have coffee? Yes, you can have black coffee, water, and plain steeped tea.

Can I add cream/sugar/milk in my coffee? The goal of fasting is to not add calories, so the answer is no, you should not add anything to your coffee. However, I have heard of cases in which intermittent fasters add less than 50 calories to their coffee and they have claimed to still be successful with intermittent fasting; I have heard that it does not affect their fasted state, but keep in mind all individuals are not created equal. I would not recommend adding anything to your coffee, but if adding something to your coffee still makes this a good change for the goal you have for yourself then give it a try.

Does intermittent fasting work well with veganism, paleo, keto, vegetarianism, or any other styles of eating? Yes, the beauty of intermittent fasting is that it can be combined with any style of eating unless otherwise directed by a medical professional. You can turn your style of eating into the 16:8 method with ease, as this change does not restrict or state the style/types of food you eat, it is specifically based on the timing of your eating.

Is there an alternative to the 16:8 method if I cannot initially fast 16 hours and want to work my way up to 16? Yes, especially for women, it is recommended that if women cannot or are not willing to do a 16 hour fast, they can start with a 14-hour fasting window and 10-hour feeding window. This is recommended for women, but men can start here if needed. Once the 14 hours is mastered, you can then work your way up to the 16:8 method.

Can I have a cheat meal? You can technically eat what you want when intermittent fasting, there are no food group restrictions. There is no cheat meal to have, unless you have decided that you have put yourself on some type of restrictive meals/foods to not indulge in, if so, then yes, but I recommend to always eat in moderation.

What are some healthy snack foods to eat on the go during my feeding window? Pepperoni slices, fruit, veggie tray, Skinny Pop popcorn individual bags (unless you will always measure the servings before consuming), turkey/beef jerky, individual peanut butter cups, whole grain cereal, almond milk, eggs, rice cakes, nuts (individual bags), hummus, and more.

I am too hungry during my fasting window, what should I do? Be patient and wait for your body to adapt to this change. This may take some time, for some it occurs fast, for others it may take a week or so, but this depends on how you were eating before you began this lifestyle. According to Collier in 2013, your body is still adjusting to how it was functioning before and is fighting you to get back to that way, as most people were eating more frequently and maybe even more meals or snacks during the day. Eventually, you will not feel this way. Eventually, you will adapt to your feeding and fasting windows and the urge to eat or the thought of starving will get easier and easier until it goes away. [11]

Why am I not losing fat faster, like other people are? It is more than likely a combination of not eating the appropriate portions when you are eating and/or not preparing to eat the right food choices. Although fat and weight loss can still happen, its more frequent and visible when the appropriate food choices and portions are selected and prepared.

How can I stay full longer? Eat more fiber and drink more water, stay hydrated.

Do I have to eat low carb? No, you can eat what you want during your feeding window. I recommend eating proportionately and choosing the healthier food options. Instead of white bread choose whole grain bread. Instead of white rice choose brown rice. Instead of anything with high fructose corn syrup, scratch it off, instead of canned fruit, eat fresh fruit.

Should I exercise in the fasted state? You can, but it is not required. It is also not recommended on heavy lifting days.

What if I am on medications and must eat with my morning medications? In this case, you would need to make your feeding window begin at whatever time you take your meds. I would recommend taking your meds as late as you can in the mornings but do get authorization of your plan from a medical professional.

Should I discuss this with my medical professional before beginning the change? Yes, you should always discuss diet changes with a medical professional before you begin.

Frequent Mistakes

People have failed due to the following frequent mistakes. Don't be one of these people, be knowledgeable and plan and think ahead.

One of the biggest mistakes beginners make is not finishing this book to the end and not taking this information seriously; basically, starting too soon, before you are prepared to start. While reading this book, it's a good idea to take notes, and jot down an individual plan while reading and sometimes doing further research during your reading. It wouldn't hurt to even read this book twice, especially if this is your first exposure to fasting, specifically intermittent fasting.

Another mistake that is made, not only with intermittent fasting but with any and most diet plans or lifestyle eating changes, is when people try to implement too many changes at once. It is not a good idea to try to become vegan and implement intermittent fasting at the same time. It is not a good idea to start working out with a trainer 4 days a week and implement intermittent fasting. It is not a good idea to start a new job with varying schedules and implement intermittent fasting at the same time. It is not a good idea to start a new medication, a new workout plan, and intermittent fasting at the same time. Not to say this is impossible, it is, but on average these are too many changes at once for a beginner.

Most of us have been taught to eat 3 good sized meals a day, breakfast, lunch, and dinner (which includes dessert) and to have snacks in between meals, so anything outside of this set up seems out of the norm. Many people are habituated to always eating something during most times of their day. Most events we host, or attend are surrounded around food and beverages, so food is always readily available. Being without food for 16 hours sounds foreign and impossible because it is not what we are accustomed too.

Intermittent fasting brings about a new idea that life is not all about eating food all the time. People are in fear of this idea at the start, which denotes negativity; they may fail in making this big of a change due to their own negative assumptions and thoughts. Do not be afraid to be hungry, you will not starve during these 16 hours, you will survive, and be successful with weight loss, better health, and weight management.

During the beginning stages of intermittent fasting, it is vital to NOT constantly watch the clock. It is recommended that you use your time wisely. Intermittent fasting will inadvertently assist you with your time management if you listen to this recommendation. While fasting, be productive, stay busy, because 16 hours of fasting is just that 16 hours of not eating. Most people will sleep the majority of the 16 hours of fasting times, but it will take time for your body AND your mind to become accustomed to not eating breakfast or not eating or drinking whatever as soon as you wake up each morning, so make sure you attempt to stay busy and never get too much in your heard or get bored.

Some people are familiar with eating mostly junk foods. No nutrients, minerals, vitamins, or any form of a balanced meal. Sugar cravings, addictions, and food obsessiveness for these people will be one of your hardest challenges. A good way to counterbalance this is to not purchase sugary unhealthy foods to be stored near you, especially during the beginning stages of intermittent fasting. We are accustomed to snacking all the time, snacking is allowed during the feeding windows, but it is recommended to make better snack options, choose fruit, not donuts, choose whole grain cereal instead of Frosted Flakes, choose nuts over candy bars.

Your body needs to be hydrated always. Sometimes your body sends your brain signals that it's hungry when you are not physically hungry, you are instead thirsty and needing liquid intake. A major mistake is not drinking an adequate amount of water daily. To assist with making water intake routine, people can start each meal with an 8 oz glass of water, drink steeped tea during either fasting or feeding times (both are acceptable), start the morning with a glass of lemon water, and/or during the feeding windows infuse water with fruits, mints, and more.

Lastly, but in no way least of the mistakes made by beginners is the idea that you don't need to choose your foods wisely. Yes, you can eat your favorite foods, yes you can still eat out at restaurants with your families, yes you can still attend social events which includes a buffet and more, but it is recommended to choose healthier options, use portion control, and read food labels if possible; basically, make smart choices to ensure you have optimal results while intermittent fasting. There is no diet or way of eating in which you can lose weight or maintain weight with no regard to calorie intake, calories count no matter what diet or way of eating you are following. Intermittent fasting is no different, you cannot get away with excessive calorie intake.

10-Day Intermittent Fasting Routine

Described below is a sample 10-day intermittent fasting routine that can be used to help you create your own intermittent fasting daily routine schedule. This will include a fasting window to include sleeping times, feeding windows, meal options with brand name recommendations in parentheses, workout plans, and more. This sample will also include varying days in life that are not as routine to illustrate how to, even with unplanned days, intermittent fasting can still be an accomplished lifestyle for most.

Time to Decide

In my personal experience and with my research, a good starting feeding window for the 16:8 method is either 11:00 AM -7:00 PM OR from 12:00 PM -8:00 PM For the purposes of creating a 10-day sample for intermittent fasting beginners, I will use the 11:00 AM -7:00 PM feeding window for this sample. With a feeding window of 11:00 AM -7:00 PM, the fasting window is then 7:00 PM - 11:00 AM The fasting time is again the time in which you do not ingest any calories. The fasting window should go by fast since the average person will be sleeping at least 6-8 hours of the fasting window hours.

Day One

5:00 AM Gulp down 16 oz of water to awaken your system. This should be your first intake each morning.

5:30 -6:30 AM High-intensity workout like jump roping, yoga, meditation, and/or some form of physical activity. This is when you give yourself a good pep talk to endure the day. The more intense the workout the more your body will be seeking food immediately after your workout, to counterbalance this try to get as much water as possible down during your workout to trick your body into thinking you are full already.

7:00 AM Drink an 8 oz warm cup of lemon water and/or a cup of steeped tea. Tea has good antioxidants that helps the body's ability to burn more fat for fuel. Warm lemon water aids food digestion as a natural flush.

8:00 AM Drink an 8 oz cup of black coffee

9:00 AM – 11:00 AM Start work. Stay busy. Be productive. Do not get bored or be lazy. Usually, beginners will start intermittent fasting on a Sunday or Monday out of habit of trying and starting many diets previously. It's a good day, especially since its day one, the most difficult day, to meal plan and prep. Review recipes online and decide on 2-3 meals that can be planned and prepped for consumption during the rest of the week. Make a food list of items you need to pick up from the store before heading home today. This will keep you busy for a while. You will need food items for at least 3 different meal options that can be eaten as lunch or dinner, you will need some snack items and drink options.

11:00 AM First meal. This is your new norm, this is what will be known as your breakfast time:

- 2 turkey sausage patties or links (Butterball), or a few slices of bacon,
- 2 scrambled eggs, an egg while, cooked in unrefined coconut oil with spinach leaves, diced onion, tomatoes, green peppers, and turkey bacon bits,
- a protein shake (Vega) mixed with unsweetened original almond milk,
- a bottle or 2 of water

1:30 PM Fruit Time: Watermelon or Melon slices, with a glass of water

3:00 PM A serving of turkey or beef jerky and a can of sparkling water (Bubly). Some sparkling waters have artificial sweeteners, and some don't, Bubly does not. Try to choose all food and drink options that include natural ingredients mostly or all the time.

Stop by the store and pick up the items from your list. While shopping you will need maybe 2 meat options, about 4 side options (preferably fresh vegetables), waters, coffee, tea, and sparkling waters. Also, pick up other items that are healthy snacks to consume during your feeding windows between meals. Some recommended staple snack items are as follows: Fruit, veggie tray, Skinny Pop popcorn individual bags (unless you will always measure the servings before consuming), turkey/beef jerky, individual peanut butter cups, whole grain cereal, almond milk, eggs, rice cakes, nuts (individual bags), hummus, and more.

Meal prep by cooking your dinner for tonight and cooking the 2-3 meals you shopped for. Once you have cooked all the meals, use containers to package all the meals up and store in the refrigerator. If you do not have good Tupperware containers that hold a full dinner and/or lunch, it is a good idea to purchase good reusable containers and to have enough for at least 5 days. You can also use small ziplock or sandwich bags to bag up healthy snack options to always have with you when you are on the go. Go ahead and pack your lunch bag for tomorrow.

6:00 PM Final meal. 6 oz boneless skinless chicken breast seasoned and cooked in an electric skillet, with a serving of broccoli and cauliflower mix, over a small bed of brown rice, with a 16 oz bottle of water and a serving of Skinny Pop popcorn. Skinny Pop Popcorn is a favorite item because you can have 3.5 cups at a low carb, calorie, and sugar count, so it is well worth it.

7:00 PM Feeding window has closed. If you get hungry before bed drink a cup of steeped green tea with freshly squeezed lemon juice to help with fat burning during your fasting window.

Day Two & Three

5:00 AM Gulp down 16 oz of water to awaken your system

5:30 -6:30 AM High-intensity workout DVD. If you are a person who doesn't have a gym membership and doesn't want to invest in one or a trainer, you can purchase low-cost DVDs to use for exercise. Also, if you have a smart TV, you can download the YouTube app and use the many free videos available to workout in the comfort of your own home. You could also use empty space in your house or apartment to start purchasing items to have a small workout room or section in your home. Drink plenty of water.

7:00 AM Drink a warm cup of lemon water and/or a cup of steeped tea

8:00 AM Drink a cup of black coffee

9:00 AM – 11:00 AM Start work. If you get bored during this time, search the internet for Intermittent fasting transformations to pass the time, or before and after pictures, or just doing more research on intermittent fasting. Learning more and seeing results, real results will inspire you and keep you motivated, as your body works to make this a habit.

11:00 AM First meal. Eat one of your meal prepped meals, as such:

- 4 oz boneless skinless chicken breast seasoned with onions, scallions, parsley, and cilantro, topped with a hint of honey,
- Salad: Made with Spinach and Arugula as the base, 2 cut up boiled eggs, banana peppers, green peppers, onions, broccoli, carrots, bacon bits, dressed with a homemade oil and vinegar mix. Using oil and vinegar as a salad dressing saves calories for something else and adds good fats to your diet,
- a protein shake (Vega) mixed with almond milk, peanut butter, cocoa powder, half of a banana, and kale and spinach leaves
- a bottle of water or two

1:30 PM Fruit Time: A green apple with an individual cup of peanut butter, with a glass of water

3:00 PM A serving of whole grain cereal, almond milk, with cut up fresh strawberries and raspberries and a can of sparkling water (Bubly)

4:30 PM An individual bag of Emeralds cocoa dusted almonds and a handful of cashews

6:00 PM Final meal. Eat one of your meal prepped meals, as such: 6 oz wild caught lemon cream-based salmon seasoned and cooked in an electric skillet, with a serving of homemade mashed cauliflower, and a small serving of black beans, with a 16 oz bottle of water and a rice cake topped with almond butter and sliced blueberries and raspberries on top

7:00 PM Feeding window has closed. If you get hungry before bed drink a cup of steeped chamomile and lavender tea to help you rest easy tonight.

Day Four (w/ Unplanned Events)

5:00 AM Gulp down 16 oz of water to awaken your system, you could always start with more than 16 oz if your body can drink that much that early

5:30 -6:30 AM Weight training, yoga, meditation, and/or some form of physical activity. Drink plenty of water, during and after your workout to stay hydrated and avoid too much of an appetite this early.

7:00 AM Drink a warm cup of lemon water and/or a cup of steeped tea

8:00 AM Today it is your colleague's birthday and your superior calls you and ask you to stop and pick up breakfast for your department (this is an unplanned event). Choose the place with your favorite coffee and buy them breakfast (to include some fruit and whole grain options) and a jug of coffee. Your feeding window has NOT started so all you will have is a black cup of coffee and enjoy the time with your co-workers. Before everything is gone, put aside a plate of fruit and a not so sugary whole grain option for you to eat later.

9:00 AM – 11:00 AM Start work.

11:00 AM First meal. Here you can insert the breakfast you set aside for yourself this morning, which could include:

- 1 whole grain bagel with one side topped with a thin layer of cream cheese
- The plate of mixed fruit and a bag of nuts that you brought from home in your lunch bag
- And another option from your lunch box, maybe your protein shake that was prepared at home
- a bottle of water

1:30 PM a hand full of mixed nuts, string cheese, and 2 slices of rolled up turkey, with 2 glasses of water

3:00 PM A pack of raisins and a can of sparkling water (Bubly)

Unplanned event: It has now been decided that your team will leave work and head to the local bar for happy hour, with traffic you will get to the bar around 5 PM

5:00 PM If you drink it is best practice to drink liquor straight with maybe squeezes of fresh lime or lemon juice. Stop consuming additives such as agave, syrups, pre-mixed drinks, etc. Ask for a double tequila with fresh lime juice on the rocks, you can maybe have 2 of these, depending on your tolerance. Your co-workers order many appetizers to share, mostly pub food, have a bite of maybe 1 or 2 options (if you cannot totally resist) then stop and either order your food at this point OR head home to eat your already prepared food.

6:00 PM You have had 2 drinks, 2 slices of Bruschetta, 2 fried wings plain no sauce. You now decide to order and eat dinner while you are here since with traffic you won't make it home before your feeding window closes. Order like the following:

- Lettuce wrapped applewood smoked bacon burger, add a fried egg, with slices of avocado
- And a side salad instead of fries, dressed with Italian dressing
- Have a cup of black coffee before you head home

7:00 PM Feeding window has closed. If you get hungry before bed drink a cup of steeped chai tea

Day Five

5:00 AM Gulp down 16 oz of water to awaken your system

5:30 -6:30 AM if the weather is acceptable, go for a light walk/run to meditate and get physical activity at the same time. If you have a friend to join you that would be even better. This is a good time to discuss your changes so far with someone else.

7:00 AM You are exhausted and did not sleep well, drink a cup of black coffee now

8:00 AM You are still not all the way woke and/or being as productive as you would like this morning, drink another cup of black coffee

9:00 AM – 11:00 AM Start work.

11:00 AM First meal. Lunch is being served at work (Unplanned Event). Taco Day:

- Make a huge taco salad to include: lettuce, chicken and steak, black and pinto beans, sour cream, cheese, guacamole, and salsa (I say huge so you can not feel bad for excluding taco shells or tortillas)
- a bottle of fruit infused water that you prepped and brought from home

- They also brought dessert: Have a mini cupcake, you deserve it

1:30 PM Drink a cup of steeped tea with freshly squeezed lemon juice

3:00 PM A box of raisins and a handful of nuts

6:00 PM As soon as you get home, you are still so exhausted from the week you crash for a nap, which turned into you being sleep for hours (unplanned event).

9:15 PM When you wake up you realize you did not have dinner and are starving, but your feeding window has closed. Drink a cup of black decaf coffee and immediately go back to sleep.

There is a lesson in NOT having that last meal, so always be sure even if it's not a big meal you eat something before that window closes.

Day Six

5:00 AM Gulp down 16 oz of water to awaken your system

5:30 -6:30 AM You are starving because unfortunately you did not have dinner last night, so you drink a cup of black coffee early to try to fight off any unwanted appetite spikes

7:00 AM Drink the second cup of black coffee and scout the internet for intermittent fasting transformations to include real pictures of before and after results and the stories of these people

8:00 AM Force drink more water and sip a cup of hot lemon water. Try to always make sure you are using freshly squeezed lemon juice, or you can purchase the lemon juice, not from concentrate in some stores

9:00 AM – 11:00 AM Start work. Here you must stay busy, keep your mind off food, otherwise you will fail and give into temptation, as this is a long fast that you anticipated due to you not having dinner last night. Keep in mind that you will not die, some people fast for days. Some people don't eat for days because they don't have food to eat, they survive and so will you. Stay in the fight

11:00 AM First meal. Turkey burger on whole wheat pita bread, with romaine lettuce, tomatoes, mayo, mustard, and a slice of swiss cheese. A serving of BBQ kettle cooked chips, a bottle of water, and two pickle spears

1:30 PM Drink a cup of steeped tea

3:00 PM Eat 2 cups of sugar-free Jell-O

5:00 PM A bag of skinny pop and a Vega protein shake, followed by a bottle of water

6:35 PM Final meal. Have a bowl of homemade ravioli. A side salad to include spinach and romaine as the base, onions, green peppers, diced eggs, diced tomatoes, dressed with zesty Italian dressing. Dessert could be 2 scoops of dairy-free Ben and Jerrys ice-cream with a bowl of strawberries. Yes, Ben and Jerrys offers about 7 dairy-free ice cream pints, they are delicious, to say the least

7:00 PM Your feeding window has closed.

Day Seven (Weekend Plans)

9:00 AM – 10:30 AM It's the weekend, which means no work for you, so you slept in this morning. At your wake up, you awake your system with 16 oz of water. Complete one hour of weight training and a light jog on the treadmill. It is also a good time to meditate and realize you have survived 7 days of intermittent fasting.

11:00 AM First meal. 2 scrambled eggs and piece of whole grain toast. You eat light because today you are headed to a local festival that will be filled with food vendors and entertainment.

3:00 PM – 6:15 PM Cajun inspired lettuce wrapped chicken wrap, with curly fries, and water to drink. 3 straight liquor drinks mixed with lime juice, and 2 corona light bottled beers

6:15 PM 2 servings of BBQ Pulled Pork with the top slice of the bun only, with 2 small corn on the cobbs with butter, and a water to drink

7:00 PM Feeding window has closed.

9:30 PM All of your friends agree to stop and eat at a diner to finish the evening (unplanned event). You order a black decaf coffee and call it a night.

Day Eight

5:00 AM Gulp down 16 oz of water to awaken your system

5:30 -6:30 AM Meditation. Drink plenty of water.

7:00 AM Drink a warm cup of lemon water and/or a cup of steeped tea

8:00 AM Drink a cup of black coffee

9:00 AM – 11:00 AM Start work.

11:00 AM First meal.

- A Boneless, Skinless 5 oz Chicken breast, Salad Greens, Apple, and Half an Avocado
- One fruit filled cup of dairy-free yogurt, and an individual bag of nuts

1:30 PM A Can of Tuna, Apple, and 1tbs of olive oil

3:00 PM 2 individual bag of Emeralds cocoa dusted almonds

6:00 PM Final meal. Eat one of your meal prepped meals, as such:

- A serving of brown rice, spinach, and mixed vegetable medley stir fry, with ground chicken meatballs and tomato sauce, sprinkled with a little fresh parmesan cheese.
- Three or fewer cookies of your choice, depending on the food label serving size

7:00 PM Feeding window has closed. If you get hungry before bed drink a cup of steeped chamomile and lavender tea to help you rest easy tonight.

Day Nine

5:00 AM Gulp down 16 oz of water to awaken your system

5:30 -6:30 AM Hot yoga with friends. Drink plenty of water.

7:00 AM Drink a warm cup of lemon water and/or a cup of steeped tea with freshly squeezed lemon juice

8:00 AM Drink a cup of black coffee

9:00 AM – 11:00 AM Start work

11:00 AM First meal.

- 4 strips of bacon
- 3 scrambled eggs
- Whole grain toast topped with grape jelly

- Half an avocado and few slices of fresh tomatoes

1:30 PM Bowl of mixed fruit and yogurt

3:00 PM Starbucks Hot Vanilla Latte with almond milk, sugar-free vanilla, 2 Splenda, and a blueberry scone that you could not resist

6:00 PM Final meal.

- 2 Packs of Sweet and Spicy tuna on an Ole Xtreme wrap with lettuce, mayo, and tomato. Three or fewer cookies of your choice, depending on the food label serving size

7:00 PM Feeding window has closed.

Day Ten

5:00 AM Gulp down 16 oz of water to awaken your system

5:30 -6:30 AM Free group trainer session with friends. Drink plenty of water. These sessions usually burn more calories, as instead of making up your own routine, you are working with a professional who knows how to get the burn out of you

7:00 AM Drink a warm cup of lemon water and/or a cup of steeped tea to stay as hydrated as possible, because usually, trainer sessions are intense, like boot camps

8:00 AM Drink a cup of black coffee

9:00 AM – 11:00 AM Start work.

11:00 AM First meal.

- 4 strips of bacon
- An omelet to include: 2 eggs, 2 egg whites, spinach, kale, onions, red and green peppers, broccoli, and fresh tomatoes

- Half of a whole grain croissant with grape jelly
- Half an avocado

1:30 PM Bowl of mixed fruit, yogurt, and a handful of cashew nuts

3:00 PM Starbucks Iced Vanilla Latte with almond milk, sugar-free vanilla, 2 Splenda, heavy cream, and 2 chocolate chip cookies

6:00 PM Final meal.

- Pulled chicken tortilla soup
- 2 fried avocado taco's
- Chicken tinga burrito
- A serving of grilled shrimp on the side

7:00 PM Feeding window has closed.

Changing it Up

How to Turn Any Diet into the 16:8 Method

The 16:8 Intermittent Fasting Method can work well with any other diet or way of eating you are already on. Most other diets are geared around restricting certain food groups or food with certain ingredients, but not intermittent fasting. Intermittent fasting does not restrict any food group, it is created this way, so you can eat your favorite foods, as long as they are eaten within the designated feeding window, and as long as you are fasting, during the designated fasting window

For those who are vegan, vegetarian, paleo, pescatarian, etc., you can still exclude what you want and still intermittent fast. To do this, eat the same way you are eating now, but these foods must be eaten within your feeding window, and you must fast within your fasting window. Nothing else must change, only the timing of your eating. For those who are low carbers, keto, weight watchers, gluten free, grain free, etc., you can still exclude what you want and include only what is allowed and still intermittent fast. To do this, you eat the same foods, drink the same drinks, and exclude what is required, you just only eat during your feeding window, and fast only during your fasting window.

An intermittent fasting vegan could have a feeding window of 10 AM-6 PM. With this you can have a vegan meal at 10 AM, Vegan snacks at 1 PM, Vegan Shake at 3 PM, and your last Vegan Meal at 5:35 PM. This illustrates that you can still be vegan and intermittent fast. This is only an example for vegans, but others can use this same plan, others like paleo eaters, vegetarians, dairy free people, gluten free people, and more.

An intermittent fasting person who is also gluten and dairy free as a consequence of health issues, also works over night as a nurse, this person feeding window may be from 11 PM to 7 AM. With this feeding window and way of eating he/she may have 3 portioned meals at 11 PM, 2 AM, and 6:30 AM, all while ensuring their meals are dairy and gluten free. As you can see, their way of eating and not eating did not have to change, only the timing of eating these meals.

An intermittent fasting keto person could increase their fats, proteins, and dairy as keto people do, as long as they are only eating during that feeding window. This persons feeding window could be from 9 AM to 5 PM. This person could have a LCHF (low carb high fat) meal at 9 AM and 4PM and the appropriate keto snacks in between.

Time management is the principal to be successful with intermittent fasting. You can exclude food groups that you want, you can include food groups that you want, you can restrict your carbs, you can restrict your calories, you can exercise or not exercise, and still be successful with intermittent fasting. The uniqueness of intermittent fasting makes it even more amazing than any other way of eating. The USDA recommends NOT restricting important food groups, so everyone should be willing to at least try it once or twice, if needed.

The Intermittent Fasting Lifestyle

Monitor & Assess Progress

If you are starting intermittent fasting to not only improve your health, but to also lose weight it is very important to take your initial weight, take measurements, and take pictures before you begin.

Scale Weigh-Ins

The morning of day 1 it is important to get on the scale either nude or in very little clothes. It is important to weigh yourself before eating or drinking anything. Choose a time and weigh yourself, this will be known as your starting weight. It is important that you not only weigh yourself but to also write this number down and/or enter it into your phone or an app that you are using to keep track of your progress. I think it's better for you to write it down in a journal along the way so you can see your progress in real time side by side.

It may also be a good idea to calculate your Body Mass Index (BMI) and your Body Fat Percentage, there are apps to calculate both, or a simple google search can result in free calculators to get this information. To prevent my scale victories from being non-victories, I choose the same day and time to weigh myself, once a week, only once a week. While intermittent fasting, you will lose inches faster than you will lose pounds from the scale, it is very important that you understand that, so that you don't get discouraged and quit. Therefore, I recommend to not only weigh yourself but to also take measurements and pictures to always see what progress you have made.

Measurement Tracking

The morning of day 1 it is important to take your measurements. You will need to buy a measuring tape to have on hand. I purchased one in my favorite color to make me feel better about myself while taking the measurements. It is important to measure yourself before eating or drinking anything. Choose a time and measure yourself, this will be known as your starting measurements. It is important that you not only measure yourself but to also write these numbers down and/or enter it into your phone or an app that you are using to keep track of your progress. I think it's better for you to write it down in a journal along the way so you can see your progress in real time side by side.

I usually take the following measurements: neck circumference, waist, hips, arms, thigh, bust, belly pouch, and calf. You can measure more or less. I take 3 separate measurements from my waist and stomach area, because feel like its 3 separate body parts. I take measurements at the same time each day and week that I weigh myself.

Before & After

The morning of day 1 it is important to take before pictures, so you have proof of how you looked on day 1. It is important to take your pictures before eating or drinking anything. Choose a time and get used to taking these pictures yourself, as someone may not always be around to help you with this (the same thing for your measurements, do this yourself), this will be known as your before picture.

I usually take pictures from all angles: front, back, both sides, one with a flexed muscle, etc., whichever pictures you decide to take do those same pictures each time you take pictures. This along with how my clothes fit is the tell all of what is really progressing and what is not or still needs work. Once, I have my pictures taken, I then use different apps to create collages to see the progress of the latest picture with the newest picture. I spend hours reviewing every inch of my body on these pictures to make sure I see all my victories. This is the best way to track your weight loss progress.

Hacks to Success

There are many principal tips and tricks that I use till this day to continue to ensure my success. While intermittent fasting is all about the timing of your meals and fasting, it can be so much more if you decide to use all the resources available to you to keep it exciting, continue to learn new things, be creative, be consistent and prepare and be prepared always. Intermittent fasting along with the hacks discussed below will change your weight and your life forever.

Sharing is Caring

I am not certain if this will help anyone other than myself or not, but it did help and is still helping me. I have learned that I am best at all things in life when I am helping others along the way. I have been sharing my knowledge with people day in and day and have become a coach of intermittent fasting to many. By encouraging others, I have simultaneously helped myself, because it's a shame to teach what you can't follow right? I won't be that type of coach. I practice what I am teaching. Me writing this book has helped me learn that I know so much about this topic, which is why I have been so much more successful this time around.

I gain so much pleasure from my social media followers interest in my story and growth. I have so much respect from my coworkers and friends and they all ask so much questions about IF, so literally this is all I talk about, which is fine by me, it holds me accountable. I don't want to let myself down to include a lot of people who are seamlessly watching me out of the corner of their eyes. I am helping someone else with this knowledge, which helps me.

Apps to Download

Pinterest is such a good resource to use when it comes to planning meals to keep eating the healthier way. This app includes links to recipes, grocery lists, meal idea, how to prep these meals, and more. YouTube, of course, is a great resource to review other people's struggles, peaks, and pits, before and after pictures, to hear their stories, to help you stay motivated and understand that most of what you go through while attempting to make this a habit, others have gone through the same things. MyFitnessPal's blog and community sections of its app is another great resource to use to join communities that are specific to intermittent fasting and all its components

These are good apps to have downloaded on your mobile device, iPad, or tablet. Using all your free time on these apps should be your new hobby instead of scrolling on your social media, especially since everything you see and hear will contribute to the success of making intermittent fasting a hobby.

Food Delivery Services

Some people decide that Meal Planning and Meal Prep is just not a realistic lifestyle for them. They may live a busier life than average, have a big active family, hate to cook, can't cook, don't want to cook, hate shopping, not creative, and more reasons. These people may choose to use a meal planning/prep or food delivery service to assist them with their meals.

Sometimes this can be costly, sometimes it may be affordable, but what it is, is convenient and by using this service you are still preparing in advance for what life throws at you during this change. You are still choosing healthier options, and being creative in what you eat.

Journaling

This lifestyle change will change your life forever. One day you will have changed so much that you may want to share your journey with others. If you decide to share, what better way to share than to go back and see how you felt each day or a few days. It is best practice to journal while you go through this journey. Journaling can be helpful in discovering what your negative triggers are, tracking your weight and measurement progress, tracking your feelings towards food, tracking your growth toward meal planning and food shopping and eating out and chosen food options, tracking your every step along the way. Your first journal entry should note why you are doing IF and explain your goals.

Sometimes people go as far as to go back to school for nutrition, or to be a trainer, life coach, and more, this journal will only assist you in tracking it all in real time. Your journal could be the road to success for someone or some other people who feel as though you once felt. This can also help you when you have those hard days and want to give up, you can read back and know that I was feeling like this once before and overcame it so surely, I can again. Journaling can only help you on this journey, it is best practice for success.

Family Lifestyle Change

I wouldn't recommend making a drastic change, but after a few days maybe a week it's a good idea to start your family and sometimes even the company you keep around you to start eating what you eat and when you eat. If you are the cook and shopper in your house, this will be a better use of your time. You will only have to meal plan once, shop once, and cook a few meals that will feed everyone for a couple of days. Hopefully, this gives you more time during the week to add in exercise if you don't, or if you do maybe a second workout, or maybe give you a few hours of time each day to do something else you have been wanting to do, like maybe writing a book.

Brush your Teeth Earlier

Everyone should brush their teeth before bed each night. With intermittent fasting, it's better to practice brushing your teeth after your last meal. The taste of toothpaste and/or Listerine should keep you from wanting to do any further eating. This is just a mind trick, but it has been a successful helpful trick that I still use.

How to Order at Restaurants

Know the menu before you go. I repeat, know the menu before you go. Most restaurants, even fast food restaurants, have websites in which you can view their menu options. If you know what's on the menu before you go, you can be proactive in deciding what you will order as the best option for you. Have a few staple times that most restaurants offer: grilled salmon, chicken breast, shrimp, any seafood, fried chicken wings no breading or sauce, burgers wrapped in lettuce, salads, and more.

Most restaurants DO NOT serve appropriate portions of food. This is an advertising mechanism for the restaurants, it is an effective way for them to get you to continually come back and spend money with them. I mean who wants to go to a restaurant that serves those small plate options. Most restaurants serve 2 and sometimes 3 times the portion that a person should be eating in one sitting.

To ensure you spend your money wisely but getting the food you pay for, while simultaneously ensuring that you are using good portion control, when you order at a restaurant it is good practice to go ahead and ask for a to-go plate and when your food arrives, split your food up by keeping an appropriate portion to eat now and package away the other 2 or 3 servings for later options.

Lunch Bag Prep

Every evening after dinner, clean the kitchen and prepare for the next day. This includes preparing my lunch bag for the next day. I add the following to my lunch bag each day. 2 full meals, 3-4 snacks, and 2-3 bottles of water and a sparkling water. Although most days, I eat dinner at home, what if I didn't make it home in time to eat dinner, or what if football practice goes long, what if traffic is a mess due to an accident, what if I must work late, what if, what if, what if. Always be prepared and you will be successful. I have had unplanned events, which have forced me to eat in the car, and sometimes dinner is a few healthy snacks because I didn't have my meal with me. Be prepared.

How to Deal with Unplanned Events

Although unplanned life events occur, sometimes 3-4 times a week, as an intermittent faster you still need to have a plan for the unplanned. Always have that lunch box/bag with you as previously mentioned. Know a few staple food options that are your go-to food options when you are on the go and don't have your own available food options. Think before you eat always.

Peer pressure is real, especially at social events, be sure to have a serious conversation with family and friends so they know you are serious and that they should not offer you items when it is not your feeding window and that your new lifestyle is not a joking matter and that you would appreciate they take it as an important part of your life. Make good decisions and be proud of those decisions that you make. Every now and then, I change my feeding windows for social events. I sometimes fast longer so that I can push my feeding window back to be able to attend social events and have dinner and drinks with family and friends.

Buy in Bulk

You may be thinking how is buying in buck related to intermittent fasting. It is vital for beginner and sometimes long time intermittent fasters to always have food on hand to accommodate any cravings and their feeding windows. It is best practice to buy favorite snack foods in bulk if available. When you buy these items in bulk you can then use small ziplock and/or sandwich bags to create your own individual serving size (according to the food label) baggies to keep in your car, purse, backpack, at school, at work, in your gym bag, in your lunch box or bag, and more.

It saves you money to buy in bulk than to buy individual items already prepackage, companies charge more for convenience, so when you buy prepackaged small cute individually packaged items it costs more than buying in bulk and doing this yourself. This also ensures that you are only having a serving or 2 according to the food label. This also saves you from not being prepared and eating unplanned food items.

Consistent Routine

Appetite is trainable because it is driven by routine. Our bodies know and learn our routines, we are usually hungry when we expect to be hungry, not necessarily when we are physically hunger, again it could be that we are bored or need fluids. Practice makes perfect, right? Fasting is a skill that with intermittent fasting you are trying to advance this skill.

Best practice would be at least start with a good routined new life as you endure this lifestyle change. That means set your alarm and wake to start most days at the same time, specifically during the week to start. Eat your first meal and 2nd meal at the same times, you can have your snacks at whatever time during the feeding window. It is also best practice to workout at the same time of the day most days and take measurements, pictures, and weigh yourself on these same days. Meal plan the week before you will shop and cook the meals. Then shop on the same day, and cook and prep the meals on the same day so you start the week always with good habits.

Setbacks

Setbacks are sometimes inevitable when it comes to any type of life change, intermittent fasting is no different. Setbacks can include general fasting knowledge, lack of discipline, willpower, self-control, fear of missing out, lack of planning or procrastination, illnesses, that may or may not include medications, that prevent this type of fasting, lack of motivation, resistance to change, YOU, and much more.

YOU

You will be your biggest setback, challenge, and critic during this attempt to change. Many people have issues with confidence, self-esteem, feeling deserving, discipline, consistency, peer pressure, unawareness, and more, which ALL can contribute to YOU being your worst nightmare during this change and ultimately maybe your demise in many aspects of life.

You must realize you are the only person who can make a change in your life, and that goes for all changes you want to make. You are responsible for your own happiness and if changing your eating lifestyle is what will make you happier, then this information gives you the knowledge to be able to make this change without help from anyone else. YOU can make this change happen for YOU, and only you. You should be beginning this journal to please only you and not just for appearance purposes, but for through and through happiness and well-being.

You must believe in yourself. You must know that you are your #1 priority and must be your biggest supporter. If no one else cares, you must care enough to change your habits and be consistent in the changes you decide to make. No one should be able to derail you from making such an important change in your life.

You are responsible for your choices. This is a LIFEstyle change so if you mess up, just do better the next time, don't quit on yourself. Don't make decisions based on temporary needs or feelings, think about what you do as you do it to make decisions that are better for you overall in the future. Think about your future, do you want to be trying another diet in another 30 days? Do you still want to be in the same body with the same health in 30 days? Would you rather feel comfortable in your clothes and skin and feel healthy throughout?

Practice Makes Perfect

Getting acquainted with the process of fasting in general and testing your chosen time frames for your feeding and fasting windows can be a difficult time if you are used to eating many meals/snacks daily. Being motivated to continue to develop in this change is just as important as anything else that comes along with this change. Live each day separately, as in if something did not go to your liking one day, change your process the next until you have feeding and fasting windows that work well with your daily routine schedule. Mind over matter, you matter, so make sure your mind continues to know this fact to ensure you aren't resistant to this change.

Don't be Weak

During the initial change stage, there must be an increased amount of willpower, discipline, and self-control. You will be required to practice your self-control around others who are NOT on an intermittent fasting lifestyle. A person needs to have the willpower to refrain from ingesting calories during their fasting window. You need to have the discipline to create these time frames and stick to them, and when the feeding and/or fasting windows are broken, create consequences for yourself to ensure it does not happen again until it does not happen anymore.

Fear of Missing Out (FOMO)

Because of how you are used to living your life, sometimes you may feel like you are missing out on the fun surrounding social and/or family eating events, but consider the fact that you are making this change to perfect how you feel and how you look to ensure you are around for a long life to enjoy life. Family and friends may not be on this lifestyle and either will or will not support this change. Alcohol should be consumed in moderation. If you choose to drink alcohol, two or less daily drinks should be the max. Choose non-sugary spirits and alcohol volume dry wines to ensure you are getting the best buzz for your choice.

Holidays will more than likely be the biggest change for you and the biggest day to test you when new to this lifestyle. Holidays are all about eating and tasting everything with family and friends and making memories. Try to prepare in advance by either assisting with cooking to ensure meals are ready before/during your feeding window and choose your favorites to ensure you are satisfied and not as vulnerable after your feeding window closes. The holidays will test you.

Prepare, Don't Procrastinate

Preparation is key. Now that you have decided on your feeding window, ALWAYS, make sure you have your meals/snacks readily available during these times. Stay ahead of your schedule a day or so, to ensure you pack your meals/snacks if you will be away from home when it is time to eat those meals/snacks to ensure. Even if you plan to be home, always make sure you take at least a few snack options with your wherever you go, by preparing in this way you ensure not to ever get caught out and about for hours with nothing to eat just wasting your feeding window away.

Not Reading Labels and Controlling Portions

Although your calories are NOT restricted when intermittent fasting, eating too much of even healthy foods can lead to weight gain no matter the type of diet/lifestyle you are following. To prevent this type of setback meal plan, use portion control, be consistent with choosing the most nutritious food choices, and measure your foods to ensure you are not eating too many servings in one meal.

Nonsense from Others

There are times in life when it's better to keep your goals to yourself. Keep your goals away from negative people, specifically keep negative people away from your goals and out of your life. To be successful in many things in life, you need a support system, which does not include negative people. You need someone who can cheer you on, someone who can motivate you, someone, who may be willing to join you, someone who doesn't add to your problems by persuading you to do what is against your goals. If you have these types of people in your life, do not tell them your plan of intermittent fasting.

Many people have their own preconceived assumptions about fasting, and intermittent fasting, and usually their views are without researched knowledge and education. It is important that you understand and know myth versus facts when it comes to intermittent fasting. People who have tried all types of diets, seem to think they know them all, and they are very discouraging at times. During a lifestyle change as intermittent fasting, it is very easy to get discouraged, so stay the course and keep those people away, while you try this out yourself based on your researched facts.

Myths vs. Facts

Understanding the differences is important to your success. Myths may create too much negative space and create room for failure. Facts should educate you enough to keep you motivated and interested in proving that you can be successful with intermittent fasting. It is a myth that not eating 5-6 meals a day will ruin your metabolism and muscle mass. It is a myth that intermittent fasting causes muscle loss, encourages overeating, causes food cravings, causes nutrient deficiencies, and is unnatural and unhealthy for your body. It is a fact that intermittent fasting creates consistencies in eating habits, helps with fat loss and weight management, and promotes a healthy system. Myths are generally kept alive for financial interest.

The Dreaded Scale

Weighing yourself daily is normal for some people, especially those who have tried so many diets, fads, supplements, diet drinks, food restrictions, etc. so this won't be any different. It is normal to want to weigh yourself daily, but this is not healthy for the success of living an intermittent fasting lifestyle. Weigh yourself one day out of the week, same day, same time, same platform and place of scale, same clothes or no clothes, etc. Weighing yourself should be part of your routine. Choose a day and time and stick to it, BUT don't get too caught up on numbers.

Intermittent fasting burns fat as fuel so the scale may not move as fast as you would expect, but to counterbalance this, you will be losing continues measurements, so be sure to take your measurements and pictures of yourself from all angles. Don't let the numbers on the scale be the thing that makes you quit intermittent fasting, observe the fitting of your clothes, keep note of your measurements and look at how your numbers drop, and create grids of before and after pictures to compare your weight success.

Social Media

It's very easy to get caught up on what you see and read on social media. The many transformation stories are fabulous and sound to simple, easy, and those before and after pictures, are like heaven to your eyes. You see that one person that you are following who's before picture looks just like you currently, and you wonder. Why haven't I gotten there? Why did it only take her 3 months to look like this? What am I doing wrong? Am I doing anything right? Is my process working? Is intermittent fasting having any positive effects for me?

A million questions will enter your mind. Some people do tell their stories, but most people tell the best of their stories and not the struggle that people have usually been having for years. Don't let anything from anyone else on social media or in passing be the reason you have setbacks or quit on this new journey. You can do this.

Illnesses

Lastly, illness could be considered a potential temporary setback, or even sometimes permanent. If this occurs, please see your medical professional on advice on how to move forward with this change or not, depending on what is recommended, sometimes it may just be a change in times or a similar change.

The Lifestyle Change and Daily Routine

Creating Habits

There is a huge adaptive component needed to be successful in changing your lifestyle to include intermittent fasting. The most important aspect is learning to create a habit, being consistent regardless of what life has to offer for you. Habits are hard to create. To create a habit, write down your daily routine and stick with it. Share your daily routine with family members to ensure they know what your new routine consists of and what it does not include. Commit to at least 21 days initial to make the habits and routine stick and make it as simple as possible.

Your response to things is what creates habits. With intermittent fasting, it is critical that during your fasting windows, if you get hungry or have cravings, that you gravitate to water, coffee, and tea, this response will become an effective response to hunger, which will create a successful habit to maintain intermittent fasting.

Skipping Days

As you begin to attempt to create habits, skipping days of intermittent fasting is not effective. Once you start this change, it is critical that regardless of weekends, holidays, social events, and more that you make this routine so that your habits begin to stick. Skipping days restarts the process for your body and mind and restarting intermittent fasting continuous is NOT a habit that you are sticking too. You must be consistent. There is no positive to put your mind and/or body through this repeatedly without committing to making it a habit.

Old Habits Die Hard

Yes, they do. Eating habits are developed in your childhood. You may not realize it, but you may still be eating like a child, as your parents taught you. I was still eating all my food from my plate when I initially started intermittent fasting. By completely devouring all my food, I realized I was not eating proportionately and was always overeating, which was one of the main issues within my old eating habits. You can eat all the healthy foods you want, but if you are overeating those foods and not using portion control, you will not lose weight, nor will you maintain weight, you will continually gain weight. This was a very big win for me when I finally discovered this and acted.

Try to observe how you eat, what you eat, when you eat, what you are doing when you eat, some aspects regarding your food relationship may be done subconsciously, and only by being very observant you can take note of certain actions and start making effective changes to be successful with intermittent fasting. Kill these old habits by any means necessary, to do that observe yourself always and figure out why you are the way you are, how are you, how can you change you and your relationship with food for the better. Change your variables to make intermittent fasting work for you.

Make it Simple

To make this a simple change, decide on your feeding and fasting windows as close to your life schedule now. Create a few meals and snack options and stick to a limited list, to begin with for meal planning and shopping; don't have too many options. Too many options could make this change seem impossible when it doesn't have to be, so keep everything simple. You don't have to journal every day if you don't just automatically gravitate to it. You don't have to measure foods and meal preps all the time, do what you can when you can, don't put too much pressure on anything.

Conclusion

With our intermittent fasting approach and now the success, we, as a couple, were able to conceive naturally and have our first child. With that fact alone, intermittent fasting has changed my life forever and made me the happiest self that I could ever be. I am extremely happy I came across what is known as Intermittent Fasting. With the so much access to the world wide web, there was tons of information to educate me on this lifestyle approach; this information guided me in so many ways and assisted me with changing my eating habits to fit my lifestyle, while also making it the best life ever.

With my success with intermittent fasting, I am no longer pre-diabetic and am in the best health of my lifetime. My body fat percentage is lower, my weight is lower, my BMI (body mass index) is much lower, I can see my abs, I have toned arms and legs, my feet size even went down (she says her bra size went down as well, which too some could be a positive or negative). I feel better. I look better. I sleep better. My clothes fit me better. And I and my family are better together.

The changes I was able to make to my own life while intermittent fasting have been super rewarding. It was also a very hard change to make, it was very difficult at first, but it taught me a lot about myself, and if I put my mind to something, no matter what it is, I can make anything happen. If I can make this change, and succeed with intermittent fasting, anyone can. That anyone includes YOU. You have to choose yourself first, you have to make yourself a priority, you have to never give up on yourself, you have to know that you are worthy, you have to know that you deserve this change, you have to WANT happiness and you have to go get that happiness for yourself. No one is more responsible for your happiness and success than you are.

Happiness comes with feeling good inside and out. Happiness comes with looking good to others, as well as, yourself. Happiness comes when you realize you have made hard decisions to better your life by being consistent and sticking to those decisions. Happiness comes when you are at optimal health and everyone, includes yourself, sees a change in you for the better. Happiness is yours, if you want it. Intermittent fasting can be step one to you becoming as happy as you want to be.

To show gratitude to intermittent fasting, I continue to spread the word about this great lifestyle. I am now an author, public speaker, and now training to be a nutritionist. Presently, I am still intermittent fasting each day. I am using the same feeding and fasting times, and I eat healthier and healthier each day as I educate myself more and more. I am a lean mean fat fighting machine, that eats my favorite foods whenever I want.

References

[14] American Diabetes Association. (2015, August 13). The Best Food Choices. Retrieved from http://www.diabetes.org/food-and-fitness/weight-loss/food-choices/the-best-food-choices/

[13] American Heart Association. (2018, April 18). American Heart Association Recommendations for Physical Activity for Adults. Retrieved from http://www.heart.org/en/healthy-living/fitness/fitness-basics/aha-recs-for-physical-activity-in-adults

[10] Berkhan, Martin. (2010, April 14). The Leangains Guide. Retrieved from https://leangains.com/the-leangains-guide/

[11] Collier, R. (2013). Intermittent fasting: the science of going without. CMAJ : Canadian Medical

Association Journal, 185(9), E363–E364.

http://doi.org/10.1503/cmaj.109-4451

[7, 9] Department of Health and Human Services and U.S. Department of Agriculture. 2015-2020 Dietary Guidelines for Americans. 8th ed. December 2015. Retrieved from health.gov/dietaryguidelines/2015/resources/2015-2020_Dietary_Guidelines.pdf.

[8] Food Allergy Research and Education. (n.d.). Milk Allergy. Retrieved October 15, 2018, from https://www.foodallergy.org/common-allergens/milk

[15] Hallböök, T., Ji, S., Maudsley, S., & Martin, B. (2012). The effects of the ketogenic diet on behavior and cognition. Epilepsy Research, 100(3), 304–309. http://doi.org/10.1016/j.eplepsyres.2011.04.017

[3] Harvard T.H. Chan School of Public Health. (n.d.). *Diet Review: Intermittent Fasting for Weight Loss.* Retrieved from https://www.hsph.harvard.edu/nutritionsource/healthy-weight/diet-reviews/intermittent-fasting/

[4] Krikorian, R., Shidler, M. D., Dangelo, K., Couch, S. C., Benoit, S. C., & Clegg, D. J. (2012). Dietary ketosis enhances memory in mild cognitive impairment. Neurobiology of Aging, 33(2), 425.e19–425.e27. http://doi.org/10.1016/j.neurobiolaging.2010.10.006

[5] Longo, V. D., & Panda, S. (2016). Fasting, circadian rhythms, and time restricted feeding in healthy lifespan. Cell Metabolism, 23(6), 1048–1059. http://doi.org/10.1016/j.cmet.2016.06.001

[17] Martin, Laura J. (2016, August 22). How to read food labels. Retrieved from

https://medlineplus.gov/ency/patientinstructions/000107.htm

[12] National Institute of Diabetes and Digestive and Kidney Diseases. (n.d.). Diet and Nutrition. Retrieved October 13, 2018, from https://www.niddk.nih.gov/health-information/diet-nutrition

[1, 2, 6] Patterson, R. E., Laughlin, G. A., Sears, D. D., LaCroix, A. Z., Marinac, C., Gallo, L. C., … Villaseñor, A. (2015). INTERMITTENT FASTING AND HUMAN METABOLIC HEALTH. Journal of the Academy of Nutrition and Dietetics, 115(8), 1203–1212. http://doi.org/10.1016/j.jand.2015.02.018

[16] Tello, Monique. (2018, June 29). *Intermittent fasting: Surprising update.* Retrieved from https://www.health.harvard.edu/blog/intermittent-fasting-surprising-update-2018062914156

Disclaimer

The information contained in **"THE INTERMITTENT FASTING 16/8 LIFESTYLE"** and its components, is meant to serve as a comprehensive collection of strategies that the author of this eBook has done research about. Summaries, strategies, tips and tricks are only recommendations by the author, and reading this eBook will not guarantee that one's results will exactly mirror the author's results.

The author of this Ebook has made all reasonable efforts to provide current and accurate information for the readers of this eBook. The author and its associates will not be held liable for any unintentional errors or omissions that may be found.

The material in the Ebook may include information by third parties. Third party materials comprise of opinions expressed by their owners. As such, the author of this eBook does not assume responsibility or liability for any third party material or opinions.

The publication of third party material does not constitute the author's guarantee of any information, products, services, or opinions contained within third party material. Use of third party material does not guarantee that your results will mirror our results. Publication of such third party material is simply a recommendation and expression of the author's own opinion of that material.

Whether because of the progression of the Internet, or the unforeseen changes in company policy and editorial submission guidelines, what is stated as fact at the time of this writing may become outdated or inapplicable later.

60676175R00069

Made in the USA
Columbia, SC
16 June 2019